Finding Your Fountain of ~~Youth~~ *Life*

Walter Young with **Maire Kushner**

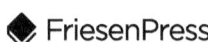

One Printers Way
Altona, MB R0G 0B0
Canada

www.friesenpress.com

Copyright © 2023 by Walter Young
First Edition — 2023

Edited by Maire Kushner

All rights reserved.

No part of this publication may be reproduced in any form, or by any means, electronic or mechanical, including photocopying, recording, or any information browsing, storage, or retrieval system, without permission in writing from FriesenPress.

ISBN
978-1-03-915053-9 (Hardcover)
978-1-03-915052-2 (Paperback)
978-1-03-915054-6 (eBook)

1. HEALTH & FITNESS, HEALTHY LIVING

Distributed to the trade by The Ingram Book Company

Table of Contents

Introduction .... *vii*
Who Is Walter Young? Why I Wrote this Book for You

Chapter 1 1
More Living in Your Life

Chapter 2 3
What Exactly Is a Fountain of Life?

Chapter 3 7
How Do I Get There? The Mode of Transportation is Your Body!

Chapter 4 13
What Will I Find? Zest for Life!

Chapter 5 15
Setting Sail!
Getting Started—Exercise and Activity 15
Getting Started—Food, Part 1 20
Getting Started—Food, Part 2 23

Chapter 6 47
Who is Your Guiding Star?

Chapter 7 49
Mentorship and Support

Chapter 8 53
Smooth Sailing and the Danger of Complacency

Chapter 9..59
Storms! Understanding Growth Through Adversity

Chapter 10..61
Which Fork in the Road? Determining If This Is What You Want

Chapter 11..65
Embracing and Accepting Your True Self

Chapter 12..73
Last Thoughts

Chapter 13..77
Land Ho! The Fountain Is a Mirror

Chapter 14..79
Epilogue

Addendum 81
Links to Complementary Articles

Acknowledgements 83

Bibliography and Citations 85

About the Author 87

About the Editor 89

Introduction

Who Is Walter Young? Why I Wrote this Book for You

I was born in Hamilton, in Southern Ontario, and lived in New York and Toronto. I was raised, like most baby boomers, to believe I would have one job, from which I would retire at sixty-five with a gold watch. Filled with a lifelong desire to help others and a drive to be independent, my approach to life was the very opposite.

From the time I left school, I found myself variously owning a hair salon, entertaining others as a stage actor in Manhattan, assisting in food prep and service, and then living in Toronto working as a personal trainer and life and fitness coach. What's next?

The inspiration for this book began with the long journey of battling my personal demons, learning important lessons, and being inspired to help others with their own challenges and life trials.

With the arrival of COVID-19, I was driven to launch the "Movement of Seniors," instilling the urge to find joy among my peers. My mantra? Don't sit at home waiting for the end of life to take you. Get up and get out!

Like most of us born in the forties, fifties, and sixties, I have lived with a self-imposed, internalized ageism. My firm belief is that this book—and any in the future—can help us understand that age is not a threat or a setback. Now, our age is our strength and our advantage. And the trick? You have to be a senior to get it!

Baby boomers know that we've been in charge of the world. And we don't wish to let that go. This Movement of Seniors is designed to inspire vitality, and the willingness and ability to grasp the joy in life. I found writing and biking and cooking and love. What will you find?

Chapter 1

More Living in Your Life

Rumours and myths of an elixir capable of restoring youth to all who drink it have persisted for generations. As early as the fourth century BC, Alexander the Great was said to have found a "river of paradise" in a site that remains famous today for its hot springs. Perhaps these are more than just hot?

As elementary school students, we marveled at Ponce de León's discovery of the so-called "Fountain of Youth," which could bestow eternal youth on all who were sufficiently fortunate to imbibe from it. Certainly, the image of his ships, sails puffed out by the wind, as he searched for the youth-granting fountain, is a legend that has remained with us. Encompassing the high adventure of the trip, exploring previously unknown territories, the entire journey held excitement and novelty never before imagined.

Is it surprising, then, that we baby boomers have seized on and embraced the present abundance of youth-extending therapies, if not life-extending treatments. We take what we can get!

So many of us may appear bionic with our mechanical shoulders, hips, or knees. We're thriving because we're enjoying the results of cardiac valve replacement, or we have a pacemaker to regulate our heartrate. Blood replacement therapies, eventual in vitro growth of replacement organs, and engineered viral gene therapies will help us find ways of overcoming all-too-common diseases that cause blindness and many other ailments.

All these futuristic solutions to the breakdown of our physical beings are on their way and will help extend our lives.

Common anti-aging cosmetics such as retinol, vitamin C, and various other topical and/or injectable treatments, as well as advances in lasers, fractional ultrasound, fat grafting or sculpting, and Botox are all (relatively) non-invasive methods of restructuring and tightening loose or sagging skin on face or body.

These methods and many more can be very useful as we try to slow the advancement of the outward indicators of our bodies aging. For many of us, this can be considered enough, but I would differ. Is it enough to let the body wear out but look good, or should the goal be to go beyond the visual and stop the rest of the aging process as well? If you think there's more to it, keep reading! Our goal here is to put as much vitality into our professed golden years as we can.

However, inasmuch as medical science is offering some solutions to aid our desire to extend our existence (or even just somewhat reduce our sagging chins!), the question of the quality of the years remaining in our lives is often overlooked.

Let me be clear, this is a book about *youthfulness and vitality*, not being young—and that's why the title is about *life*. I am by no means an expert on this. I am merely an observer and regular participant. I have seen what works for me specifically, and I also try to draw information from sources with deeper pockets and infinitely more resources than I have. I'm going to take you on a journey. That is all.

Why should you use me as your guide?

Well, let's start off with the obvious. I am one of you. I was born in the late fifties, played until I got high in high school, and started dancing. I discoed, punked, new-aged, and, like so many others, cleaned up my act in the nineties. I came into my own in the early part of this century, and have truly hit my stride since. I have turned my life around, and found a way to reclaim what I feared had been lost with the passage of years. Much has been trial by error, but thankfully, a great deal has been with the help of my self-constructed village. Do I know everything? *Not in the least!*

Allow me to hold your hand as we pass this way together.

Chapter 2

What Exactly Is a Fountain of Life?

Do I Want to Go? Why Should I Look for It?

Great questions! Sometimes, we look at the idea of changing or travelling, and immediately, a little voice says, *What will I pack? What if I don't enjoy the food? Who else is going? I might not like them! They might not like me! Who will take care of my cat?* (This final question is of particular concern to me.) Or, on a deeper level, *Who will I be if I change?* From experience, having quit drinking, and—years later—quit smoking, I was left with a fear of who I would turn into as these vices were removed. To steal from the book, *Alcoholics Anonymous*, "Would I be the hole in the doughnut?" What I know is that we will do whatever we can to talk ourselves out of making significant changes because unless where we are is unbearable, remaining at rest or just making no effort at all is easier than change.

As a gay man, trying to stay young has always been an important goal. I learned very early that there is a stigma associated with the appearance of aging. Clearly the myth of *invisible-over-forty* (or sometimes over fifty) persists. In the general public, women have faced this kind of discrimination for years—and now men are also being asked to stay young to remain relevant in the workplace. I started moisturizing in my teens and swore not to smile through my twenties (causes wrinkles, don't you know?). Despite the effects of smoking and suntanning and their correlation with aged-looking skin, here I am at sixty-five, absolutely still moisturizing as a protective measure, and finally adding sunscreen regularly.

I grew up with parents and grandparents who thought of forty as middle-aged and sixty-plus as senior—people who had tons of *stop doing that at your* *age* standards. Having dealt with internalised homophobia, I now find myself dealing with *Gerascophobia,* * internalised but also reversed into the form of ageism that finds me asking myself, "*Why are you doing that?*", "*Aren't you a little too long in the tooth for that?*", "*Act your age!*" How easy it is to lapse into letting time take its toll. Can I just fight these impulses?

*Gerascophobia: An abnormal and persistent fear of growing old. Sufferers of this fear experience undue anxiety about aging, even though they may be in good health—physically, emotionally, financially, and otherwise. They may worry about the loss of their looks, the loss of independence, inactivity after retirement, impaired mobility, the onset of disease, and the unthinkable—being confined to a nursing home. Modern society's preoccupation with youthful beauty does nothing to alleviate these fears.

Genetic Studies

New research suggests that it is possible to slow or possibly reverse aging, at least in lab mice, by undoing changes in gene activity—the same kinds of genetic modifications that take place in humans, caused by living life for many decades.

These studies add weight to the scientific argument that aging is largely a process of so-called epigenetic changes—that is, alterations that make genes either more or less active. Over the course of our lives, cell activity regulators are added to or removed from our genes. In humans, these changes can be caused by smoking, pollution, or other environmental factors, which can dial genetic activity up or down. As these changes accumulate, our muscles tend to weaken, our minds may slow down, and we become more vulnerable to disease.

A new study in lab animals suggests the possibility of reversing at least some of these genetic modifications—a process researchers think may eventually work in living humans. "Aging is something plastic that we can manipulate," says Juan Carlos Izpisua Belmonte, who has multiple advanced degrees at various international universities and is currently an expert in gene expression at The Salk Institute (named for Jonas Salk, the inventor of the polio vaccine), which facilitates his mission of daring to make dreams a reality.

The Salk Institute's internationally renowned and award-winning scientists explore the foundations of life, seeking exciting new understandings of neuroscience, genetics, immunology, plant biology, and more. The institute is an independent, non-profit organisation.

So, if we are living longer, don't we want more living life in our lives? How do you want the next twenty, thirty, or fifty years to go?

By making the decision to, at minimum explore some of the seemingly impossible possibilities that may exist, we are invoking change. This is exactly the same kind of change that will take place as we push off from the dock on our new journey. The only way to start is to start. If you've come this far, you know that the concept of this adventure is worth at least a perfunctory look.

It's not inconceivable that many of us will live to a hundred years of age, or even longer. What is the most reliable vessel we can choose that will provide us the best chance of living a long, consequential life of substance?

What kind of boat do you want to carry you on your voyage?

Chapter 3

How Do I Get There?
The Mode of Transportation is Your Body!

We have many choices to make on our journey, but the primary and most significant is how and why to maintain our ship. It's a long journey! Do you want to worry about leaking, bailing, and falling apart? Do you want to maintain your craft, a vessel of inestimable value? Our Fountain of Life is best reached with a well-preserved vessel.

What kind of boats are there? Let's examine:

The Bodybuilder

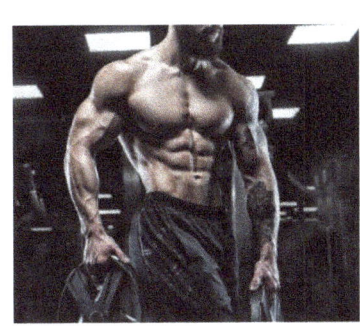
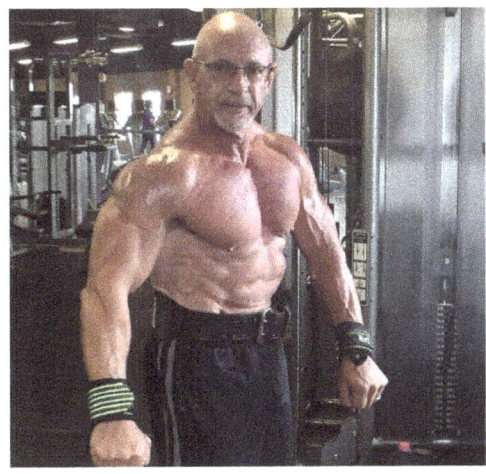

The Runners

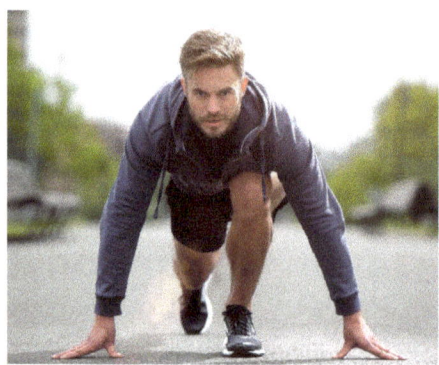
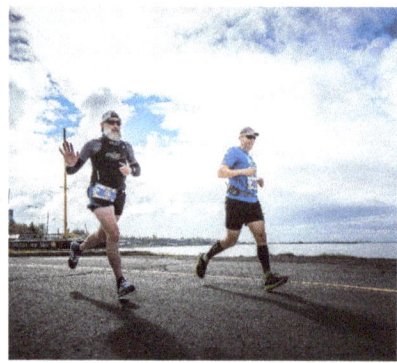

The Yoga Masters

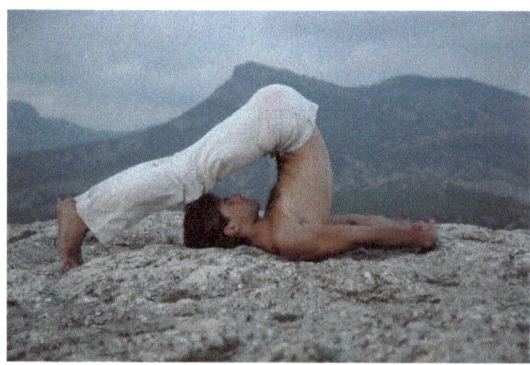
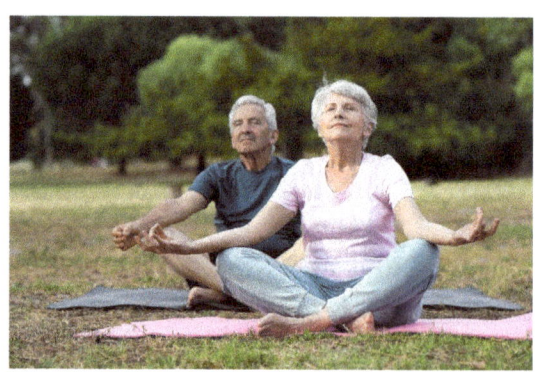

Finding your Fountain of ~~YOUTH~~ Life

The Ironman

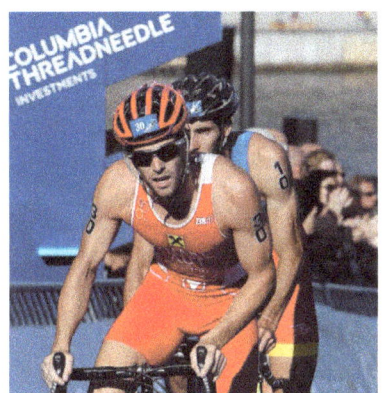
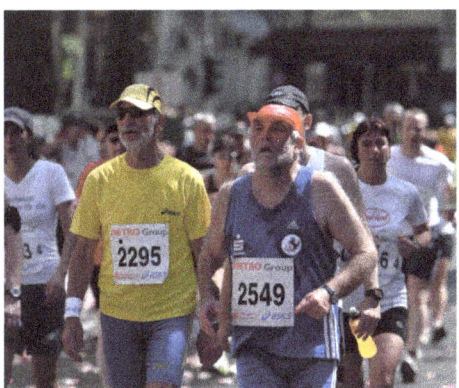

All body types are good body types. Fit bodies have different compositions, as in the examples above. The added muscle mass of the bodybuilder could hamper the speed of the runner or triathlete. The overall levels of cardiovascular health are also widely different between the various types.

As a bodybuilder, I push farther to gain and keep muscle, maintaining a specific aesthetic ideal. But a high level of cardio conditioning coupled with muscle mass should keep me going into my next century. Creating a balance between the two will give us longevity and improve our ability to perform all the foundational tasks that keep us independent.

Now, you may ask, *I am average, and I don't want to be some kind of elite athlete.*

Before we move on, let me say that it was very difficult to find average photos of a typical octogenarian—at least, those individuals not seated in an armchair. Does that mean that there aren't those who are active? Absolutely not! But it is an example of media representation. And if I may be so bold, if you are an active person over the age of sixty-five, *you are an athlete*, whether you are working out two or three times a week, swimming, biking, or engaging in other, regular, strenuous movement—perhaps even running a marathon.

It took me more than ten years of living with fitness to be able to use these words, but there is no other way to put it: I am an athlete! *Claim it*! This is as difficult for a twenty-year-old as it is for those of who've been on the planet longer. It is the best descriptor!

"Physical activity is an integral part of healthy aging. According to the US Center for Disease Control and Prevention (CDC), 16.3 percent of adults ages sixty-five to seventy-five and 9.9 percent of adults ages seventy-five and older met the aerobic and muscle-strengthening Physical Activity Guidelines for Americans in 2018, the lowest of any age group." [1]

You may be thinking a lot of things right about now, like, *My doctor says I should…* If he says, "Take it slow," he's definitely right. Life is a marathon, and smarter, more cautious behavior will portend a life without injury. If he says "Change your diet," he's also probably right. If he says "Relax, enjoy your age and take it easy", *smile and find a new doctor.*

I hear things all the time. I hear from my own doctor about how I should lose weight, because according to the charts, at my age and height, I should weigh *x*. Nothing could be farther from the truth!

I will pay attention to charts about smoking, cholesterol, and all the mitigating factors that lead to disease, but not a chart that's used to sell life insurance that says it's important to weigh a certain amount in accordance with height and age.

In fact, according to diabetes.ca:

"BMI is not used for muscle builders, long distance athletes, pregnant women, the elderly, or young children. This is because BMI does not take into account whether the weight is carried as muscle or fat, just the number. Those with a higher muscle mass, such as athletes, may have a high BMI but not be at greater health risk. Those with a lower muscle mass, such as children who have not completed their growth, or the elderly who may be losing some muscle mass, may have a lower BMI. During pregnancy… a woman's body composition changes, so using BMI is not appropriate." [2]

Because of my professions as a trainer and a body builder, I will go against the flow and try to gain weight, as it is an indicator of muscle mass. One of the most striking effects of age is the involuntary loss of this critical muscle mass, termed *sarcopenia*. Muscle mass decreases approximately 3 to 8 percent per decade after the age of thirty, and this rate of decline is even higher after the age of sixty.

The significance of a doctor's oversight cannot be denied. Important issues like blood pressure, heart functions, certain vitamin and mineral levels, blood components, etc. need to be monitored after a certain age.

But let's be honest here: with very few exceptions, maintaining a progressive level of fitness is always going to help maintain good general health and eliminate many of the underlying causes of malfunction in the above indicators. And we should maintain a level of personal responsibility, even if it means walking into the doctor's office with a list of concerns. If you don't ask, you don't know.

Chapter 4

What Will I Find? Zest for Life!

There has to be a real reason to make the type of changes we're discussing. As I've learned through the reading I've done, we are either running to something better or running from something bad; it's the pleasure/pain principle. Often, it can be a combination of both.

In my case, I'm running toward a future that is free of pain and full of the kinds of activities that will facilitate completing the joyous final chapters of my life. I have had the opportunity to view the opposite with my parents, who were both taken far too early by diseases mostly brought on by lifestyle choices. They were the reason I quit smoking, changed up my diet, and became more active, paired with the examples of others who'd had extended lives, such as my grandmother and some of my early mentors. In all honesty, it still took almost fifteen years between the loss of both of my parents and the day I smoked my last cigarette. Sometimes, these types of changes are not automatic.

Working with my clients, I frequently see that parents want to get fitter so the quality of the time spent with their children will be improved and extended. Then, it becomes the same mantra with respect to their grandchildren—to be able to play with them, pick them up, and generally participate in their lives.

Given the possibilities of the scientific extension of human lifespan, extension of the "healthspan" becomes more vital, and may just provide us with the opportunity to play with and participate in the lives of our *great*-grandchildren.

Although I was fortunate enough to have known one of my great-grandparents, believe me, we did not play together!

Let's also think about the wonders we might see with life extension. I'm a diehard optimist and having seen the first moon flight and now the possibility of Martian colonies (Holy Ray Bradbury!), I want to know where we end up. Having seen the ridiculous and unbelievable world of TV's *Star Trek* actually happening with computers, communications, health scans at our wrists, being able to tell our artificial intelligence aide to perform simple tasks in our homes, all point to a future worth seeing—and I definitely want to be here for as long as I can. Even now, I am working with an assistant who lives on the opposite side of the planet.

This does, I think, require a certain level of optimism—otherwise, what joy would we see in imagining this? So, here's the big warning:

If you think there'd be no point to living longer, thinking, *those kids won't want to spend time with some old person*, if you feel that the good old days were the best and the world is going to hell in a handbasket, that all this scientific change is not good for us, well...

SNAP OUT OF IT!!!

A closed mind closes the door to enjoyment of life.

Chapter 5

Setting Sail!

Getting Started—Exercise and Activity

OK, let's get on our way, but let's be smart about it. We're not sitting down at the piano and immediately playing a Mozart Concerto. Being forced to play piano can lead to fear and loathing of the instrument and even the concerto.

The idea I am offering you is to start slow and with an open mind. Find what turns you on—what makes it fun to get fit.

The actual activity (or activities) you choose can take as much time as your enjoyment will encompass. At the outset, I recommend something like twenty minutes a day dedicated to fitness. Somewhere in the scrolling, binge-watching, eating, drinking, and living, we all have that much time tucked away. As you find what you like, you will be drawn to devote more time to it.

Thinking a bit about my recent journey: I had, for the longest time, relied on the machines at the gym to create a level of cardio for me, forgetting how much I'd enjoyed the walks that were the early foundation of my fitness journey. With the advent of COVID-19, I returned to walking, taking photos, and letting nature instill some extra strength in me. Soon enough, I started jogging and walking (but not on hilly or rough terrain). This built into ten-kilometre runs and, thanks to a good friend, cycling. *Yahoo*!

All this has led to my newest challenge, and I am now a budding triathlete. Don't misunderstand—I'm not saying that everyone needs to follow my path—not unless you want to. What I am suggesting, though, is to get started and let yourself be led forward by your progress and your interests. You will find the journey that is best for you.

As a side note, one of my rules when walking was to not take the same route every day. So, arriving at an intersection, I would venture down a different road, including alleyways. I have discovered so many exciting pieces of graffiti art, hidden parks and gardens, architectural jewels! It fills me with gratitude. And this attitude makes my morning constitutional walk a bit more of an adventure.

Have questions?

It looks so hard to change like that—not to mention how expensive it will be! We need to examine your definitions of difficult and expensive. For example, going for a walk is not expensive, but climbing Kilimanjaro is. Starting out shouldn't cost anything, because I'm advocating a brisk walk to start the day, and that's always going to be free. As time goes on and you perhaps want to join a gym, it will cost more, but with community and fitness centres, municipally operated pools, and coupons—like on Groupon and ClassPass—that discount memberships at private gyms, inexpensive options abound.

But what's the real expense? The cost of a sedentary lifestyle is greater than the cost of fitness. Losing the ability to move, reduced cardiac capacity, high blood pressure, and obesity don't have to be part of the aging process. We can have some control over the pace of the digression of our bodies.

What's different now than when we were younger? I hope we have gained some level of sense and a degree of sensibility. Now older, assuredly, and wiser, somewhat, my *plan is to plan*. The younger version of myself would have jumped into a new business or hobby or relationship without considering the repercussions or consequences. This does not mean I won't move forward or that I'll resist a challenge. Now, though, instead of picking up the two-hundred-pound weight, I'll have a trainer demonstrate proper form and efficient, effective practice. Fools rush in, yes, but that doesn't mean that fear should prevent movement.

We're starting a long journey, one which we hope will persist for the remainder of our lives. With that in mind, we need to ensure that the vessel in which we're travelling is also going to last as long as our journey. Statistics indicate that this will be a long time, as life expectancy increases each year.

**Standing still is always easier,
until the point of change becomes impossible.**

I'd like to introduce you to the quintessential late starter: Sister Madonna Buder, also known as the Iron Nun, who completed her 390th Ironman Triathlon at eighty-nine years of age while living as a Roman Catholic religious sister. She started training  when she was fifty-two with her first triathlon, and at fifty-five, completed her first Ironman. She is now a Senior Olympian Triathlete. As she writes in her book, *The Grace to Race: The Wisdom and Inspiration of the Eighty-Year-Old World Champion Triathlete Known as the "Iron Nun,"* "I feel very blessed and very grateful to keep on going as if there were no time limits. I think it's best not to pay any attention to age, but to who you are while you are in the process of getting there."

There are many examples of those who have changed route in their fifties, sixties, and beyond, and these are the people to read about, study, and use as markers in our own lives. Life is an evolutionary process; growth and change do not stop at a fixed time.

Alan Rickman, actor, first movie at forty-six.

Julia Child, chef, and TV personality, who was fifty when she hosted her first TV show.

Martha Stewart, chef, author, and household maven was forty-one when she published her first book, Entertaining, *and forty-eight when she launched Martha Stewart Living.*

Charles Darwin, explorer, and author was fifty years old before he published On the Origin of Species *in 1859, the book that espoused the theory for which he best known today. (The Darwin Awards came much later.)*

Samuel L. Jackson, forty-six years old (and in recovery from addiction to cocaine and heroin), before he starred alongside John Travolta in Pulp Fiction.

Anna Mary Robertson Moses, American folk artist, known by her nickname Grandma Moses. She began painting in earnest at the age of seventy-eight and is often cited as an example of an individual who successfully began a career in the arts at an advanced age.

J.R.R. Tolkien, author, was forty-five when The Hobbit *was published in 1937. He is best known for the* Lord of the Rings *trilogy, which has sold over 150 million books worldwide. Tolkien is called the father of modern fantasy literature, ranked fifth in Forbes's highest earning "dead celebrity" category in 2009. His novels were even made into films, which have racked up millions at the box office.*

Finally, I'd like to introduce one of my faves, although she was not as famous. Adeline De Walt Reynolds was born during the American Civil War, in 1862. Although she'd always wanted to become an actress, due to family constraints, she did not. Adeline began her career with a lie, claiming she was twenty when only eighteen to qualify as a teacher. She fought to have pay equal to her male colleagues' and having lost that battle, left teaching. Around 1890, she graduated from the Boston Conservatory of Speech, where she was in training to become a speech therapist. Much later, when widowed with four children and studying to become a secretary, the school where she was enrolled was destroyed by the 1906 San Francisco earthquake. Talk about hard knocks!

After all her children had grown and left home, Adeline returned to school, graduating French language studies with honours from the University of California at Berkeley. She was sixty-eight and was finally able to return to her first love, taking acting classes at the Stella Adler School.

De Walt Reynolds made her film debut with a supporting role in Come Live with Me *(1941), playing the grandmother of James Stewart. Her last film was* The Ten Commandments *(1956), where she portrayed a frail, old Israelite fleeing Egypt. She played her last television role at the age of ninety-eight. At the time, she was the oldest member of the Screen Actors Guild. And here's what I love: she also made publicity stories and photos that showed her practising her fencing techniques or doing calisthenics. Fit until the end! De Walt Reynolds died on August 13, 1961, one month before her ninety-ninth birthday.*

So, if you're feeling like you are not where you want to be with your passion, whatever that may be, you still have a lot of time to create your footprint.

How Long Is Our Voyage? How Much Time Will It Take?

The answers to these questions are individual. They will depend on your own personal goals and targets. Resist the urge to compare yourself to others! This is a more than strong warning. Whenever I have compared my journey or accomplishments with someone else's, it has been used by my inner saboteur to show me that I wasn't up to some imaginary standard. Conversely, this allowed me and my inflated ego to put myself above others and get complacent about my own work. Both are detrimental to our progress. Do your best on any given day. That's it!

If you set your objectives with the constant image of improvement, and recognize your incremental achievements and victories, you will succeed. Never forget that failure is an opportunity to learn.

Another example of the senior Ironman. Meet Lew Hollander, in his eighties.

Getting Started—Food, Part 1

While this chapter is about nutrition and fuelling the boat properly, I think it's critical that I dispel some of the myths, clear some of the fog, and then examine what's real and what's imaginary or just plain trendy in the area of food.

As a trainer, it is relatively easy to get people to grasp good form while exercising. Teaching good form with diet is a much more complex matter.

Why?

There are so many diets—and by that, I mean weight loss methods, not different cultural cuisines associated with a specific race, sect, geographic area, or religion. All so-called weight loss diets are "guaranteed" to work, but what is at the core philosophy of each? What main principles applied actually help someone to lose the weight?

All diets work on two complementary premises: there will be restrictions on some types of food and the quantities of some others; and there will be decreases in the intake of calories created by these restrictions.

Currently, the most popular diets are…

The Paleo Diet: This diet emphasizes foods and beverages that would have been the only means of sustenance for humans in prehistoric and pre-agrarian times (Paleozoic Era)—fruit, vegetables, nuts, and meat. The program eliminates processed foods, as well as sugar, table salt, caffeine, legumes, and dairy. While some tubers, such as sweet potatoes, are allowed, most grains are not. By removing dairy and many carbohydrates, caloric deficit occurs and weight is lost. For some, these restrictions are not difficult to adapt to their lifestyle plan, and they find that the paleo diet is more easily sustainable than others.

The Keto Diet: The name "ketogenic" comes from ketosis, which is the body's process of turning fat into energy. A ketogenic diet stresses the consumption of natural fats and protein, such as meat, fish, and poultry, while limiting almost all carbohydrates, which will maintain the state of ketosis over a sustained period of time.

Because you feel full for a longer period of time after eating these fats and proteins, your appetite is reduced and you therefore consume fewer calories overall.

Despite the popularity of the ketogenic diet, there are plenty of myths surrounding it. This is a highly elevated version of the Paleo diet that requires adding extra fats but no extra carbs in order to create energy for the body. It is much more difficult and therefore less sustainable for most people.

There is even a subset of this diet, the Carnivore diet, which has no vegetable nutrients—only meat, eggs, and some dairy products. And this diet has a further subset that removes the dairy and eggs. Proponents speak of lowered inflammation, better energy levels and a stabilised bodyfat level.

The Ultra-Low-Fat Diet: The ultra-low-fat, or very-low-fat diet allows for no more than 10 percent of calories from fat (most acceptable guidelines suggest approximately 30 percent). It also tends to be low in protein (about 10 percent of daily calories) and very high in carbs (80 percent of daily calories). Ultra-low-fat diets are mostly plant-based, limiting your intake of animal products, such as eggs, meat, and full-fat dairy. High-fat plant foods, including extra virgin olive oil, nuts, and avocadoes, are also often restricted, even though they're generally perceived as healthy.

Again, with restriction comes caloric deficit and weight loss—perhaps a bit more with these extreme constraints, because unfortunately, the greatest benefit of fats to the eater is added flavour and mouthfeel. When flavour is removed, the desire to eat is also lessened.

Are these extreme diets sustainable? Not for most of the population.

Every diet on the planet recommends that something is removed from your regular nutritional plan—one says no carbs, one says no foods that cause inflammation, or no proteins, or even no solids (everything is pulverized in a blender/juicer). The immediate result of this is a predictable shift in your metabolism, and corresponding weight loss.

Your new diet will regulate what amount you eat. You will be instructed. You'll be sent pre-prepared food and/or you'll have to diarize all intake. You'll definitely be ingesting less than you might have before.

So, what happens? Weight loss! Great!

But then reality hits, because we're human, and have to live in the real world. No one likes to feel deprived. Even when the diet allows so-called "cheating" or "cheat days," the very concept of the word "cheat" implies something negative, something guilt-inducing. Inevitably, you'll be invited to a dinner party, have no time for a meal, or be starving—"So, let's just pull into this takeout and grab a salad." Or, "I miss my favorite food," and on and on. What happens? Negativity and guilt become components of your "diet."

What's your favorite meal? Or your desert island dish? Could you remove these permanently if they weren't an allowable item on a diet? Could you jettison a treasured holiday item. More importantly, do you want to?

I firmly believe that we need to be human and enjoy the incredible gift that is food and the pleasures of the table. Let's just not make every meal a feast.

These are just a few of the possible paths to follow if quick weight loss is your desired outcome. We won't be wasting any time with the diet of the week, or the Hollywood star's diet, or the "Cabbage Soup for a Week" diet. These may work at the outset, but they are not advisable, healthy, or sustainable.

Nutrition is *not* deprivation.

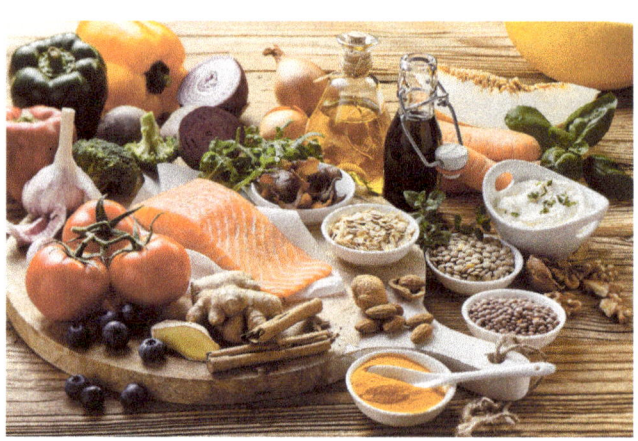

Getting Started—Food, Part 2

Put the wind in your sails!

Food is Fuel

Even if you follow the programs in part One, your body will adapt and become adjusted to the deficit in caloric intake. Then what? Plateau or worse—weight gain! No!!!

Now what?

What I want to inform you of are real, legitimate, sustainable eating habits to get us through the next twenty, thirty, or fifty years—and even beyond. What does a body need to build muscle, sustain energy, and provide us with the micronutrients we need to maintain optimum health and its benefits?

What is the 30/30/40 Rule?

This rule is a general, best-practice model I believe in. Not only will it allow you to maintain optimal metabolic maintenance. It can also act as a yardstick by which to examine the diets listed previously.

As a guiding principle, it means that my food consumption will adhere as closely as possible to ratios of 30 percent carbohydrate, 30 percent fat, and 40 percent protein. As shown below, your plate would look blue protein, green carb, red fats.

This ratio eating is also a tool by which we can improve the results specific to the needs of an individual. By removing 5 percent of both carbs and fats, my client the bodybuilder, prepping for competition, can improve on muscle-building results (in keeping with the rigours of their exercise program); whereas my marathon runner might add to the carbs and remove the added protein and fat. It allows for flexibility to suit the individual.

So, what I would really like to drive home here is the concept of the "best diet" being an impossible goal. Nutrition is not based on a set of what is allowed and what is not allowed; it is the concept and implementation of healthy eating, creating the desired results. Losing or gaining weight is not about removing an entire element from your diet or making a practice of not eating at all every second day. My job here is help you understand that there are no "perfect" diets, and you searching for that is an impossible task.

40% Protein Intake

PROTEIN

Protein is what muscles are made of.

I've already talked about muscle loss as part of the aging process. If you weigh *x*, multiply your weight in pounds by 0.36. For a fifty-year-old woman who weighs 140 pounds and who is sedentary (doesn't exercise), that translates into fifty-three grams of protein a day. Now, if you're active the amount needed to rebuild muscle has to be factored in as well. To lose weight, diets with higher amounts of protein—between 90 and 150 grams a day—are effective, and will help maintain muscle mass while losing fat, so if you're not ingesting a sufficient amount of protein and you're exercising more, loss of muscle mass will occur. Vegetarians have many excellent proteins available, and can just as easily sustain muscle growth. Once one learns how these food groups can be used for optimal protein intake, preparation and meal planning become much simpler.

Are you a vegetarian? No problem! You'll need more thought and planning to ensure that proper protein/fat/carb combinations are made. This will take some time but is worth the effort and pays many dividends.

Protein as Part of the Aging Process

Excerpt from:

"Protein for Fitness: Age Demands Greater Protein Needs"
By Denise Webb, PhD, RD
Today's Dietitian
Vol. 17, No. 4, p. 16 [3]

Studies suggest how much protein is needed for active older adults to build and maintain muscle for optimal health. Older patients need more protein than their younger counterparts.

Though greater protein needs for older individuals aren't yet reflected in the Recommended Dietary Allowances (RDAs), it's clear that not only do older people progressively lose muscle as they age, but also their physiology resists building new muscle. The muscle loss, known as sarcopenia, ranges anywhere from 0.5 to 2 percent of total muscle mass each year, starting around age fifty.

The good news is that after age fifty, getting enough high-quality protein in the diet, coupled with physical activity, can help overcome that resistance…

"The combination of resistance exercise, such as lifting weights or push-ups, and higher protein intakes appear[s] to protect muscle and strength, even during weight loss," says Donald Layman, PhD, a protein researcher and professor emeritus in the department of food science and human nutrition at the University of Illinois…

"No one has done an age-related curve of protein needs," Layman says, "but by age sixty-five, you need the combination of exercise and high-quality protein. Older adults are less efficient in using amino acids for muscle protein synthesis than are young adults. Exercise increases the efficiency of muscle protein synthesis in older adults."

What about vegetarians? Older vegetarians can achieve the higher recommended protein intake, but it requires much more planning and forethought…Vegetarians should get protein from soy products, such as tofu, soymilk, and soy yogurt; lentils; beans; nuts; and seeds.

Protein at Every Meal

While not everyone agrees, some experts believe that equally distributing protein intake over three meals during the day is just as important as getting enough protein overall. The distribution is important for maximizing the utilization of amino acids for muscle tissue synthesis… Seniors should strive for thirty grams at each meal and include protein in snacks as well. An example of a thirty-gram protein breakfast can include one scrambled egg and two Italian veggie sausage links… Breakfast can be the most neglected meal when it comes to protein, and a "tea and toast" breakfast isn't conducive to maintaining muscle health.

Senior Athletes

But what about people who stay physically active well into their sixties, seventies, and even eighties? Running, walking, cycling, hiking, even running marathons? Do they need even more protein than their less active counterparts of the same age, and how much is enough?

…Obsessing over the right proportion of protein in the diet in unnecessary, unless you're going for the gold and training hard or working toward some personal best.

30% Carbohydrate Intake

CARBOHYDRATES

There are three main types of carbohydrates:

Sugar (glucose): fruits, vegetables, milk and milk products. Types of sugars include fruit sugar (fructose), table sugar (sucrose), and milk sugar (lactose).

The umbrella chemical term for sugar is "glucose." Each type is differentiated by its source. Regardless of the type, the body can only store so much sugar calorically. Excess glucose (sugar of all types) is stored in your liver, muscles, and other cells for later use. This extra sugar ingested is converted directly to fat.

Starch: Carbohydrates (starch) are your body's main energy source.

Carbs occur naturally in vegetables, grains, and cooked dry beans and peas. They are used to fuel all of your activities, whether you're going for a jog or simply breathing. These are the key types of nutrients which can be broken down during digestion into sugars, for use as energy.

When discussing carbohydrates, it is important to differentiate between fibre and other carbs because fibre is not broken down into sugar. In fact, the body can't break it down at all.

I wouldn't be doing my job if I didn't add the downside here. The Western diet, at present, has a preponderance of carbohydrates. Have your toast, and a pastry for a snack, some kind of pasta, rice, or potatoes throughout the day. And to make it more difficult, thinking that fat is the enemy, carbohydrates are ingested to give "fat-free" foods a better taste and mouthfeel. Don't be fooled!

Fibre: Fibre is essential for optimal digestive health. Fibre is a complex carbohydrate, naturally occurring in fruits, vegetables, whole grains, and cooked dry beans and peas. In addition to the critical role it plays in our digestion, it also aids in protecting against obesity and Type 2 Diabetes. Fibre ingested passes through the body and is eliminated.

Because our bodies are unable to convert fibre to sugar, consuming fibre performs some very important tasks; it either helps waste to be removed, helps your body absorb nutrients, or actually serves as waste material keeping your digestive system functioning well.

What exactly is fibre? In addition to the foods listed above, fibre is in the seeds of berries and many fruits, the husks of grains (which we remove when producing industrial and many commercial foods), the skins of apples and other fruits, the string in the celery stick, the part of the corn that sticks between our teeth. It also is part of quinoa and unpolished rice.

These are good for you and should be eaten frequently.

One extra benefit of eating fibre is that it adds to the sense of satiety or feeling full at the dinner table. Paying attention to this sensation is critical to managing our weight, as it contributes to less overeating.

30% Fat Intake

FAT

Fat has a bad rap.

Fat is complex. Fat is not desirable as a state. Fat is important but is misconstrued as being harmful to us. In fact, humans need fat as:

- A source of energy
- A source of essential fatty acids that our bodies are unable to make on their own. Food is the usual way we acquire these fats, but supplements are a good alternative (see the section on fats to follow)
- A component of cell walls
- A way to absorb fat-soluble Vitamins, A, D, E, and K
- A way to insulate our bodies and protect our internal organs

Fat tends to be considered "bad" because it is associated with obesity, high blood pressure, heart disease, high cholesterol, and other undesirable conditions. However, certain types of fat provide protective benefits to the heart, if consumed in reasonable and suitable quantities. The key to understanding a "suitable" amount is knowing how to choose the right amount of each type of fat. Let's examine the idea of total fat and proper quantities of each.

FATS

Total Fats

The dietary reference intake (DRI) in adults is 20 to 35 percent of total calories from fat—that is, about forty-four to seventy-seven grams of fat if you are consuming two thousand calories per day. It is recommended to eat more of some types of fats, because these provide recognized health benefits. Correspondingly, we should be consuming less of other fat types because they have a negative effect on our health. Here's the recommended ratio:

- Mono-unsaturated fat: 15 to 20 percent
- Poly-unsaturated fat: 5 to 10 percent
- Saturated fat: less than 10 percent
- Trans fat: 0 percent
- Cholesterol: less than three hundred milligrams per day

Unsaturated Fats Are Mostly Good

These fats are usually liquid at room temperature, like olive oil and peanut oil, and their sources include mono-unsaturated and poly-unsaturated fats. When used in place of saturated fat, mono- and poly-unsaturated fats can help lower levels of bad cholesterol (more on this later).

Mono-unsaturated fats from plant-based sources include olive, canola, and peanut oils, nuts and nut butters, olives, and avocados.

Poly-unsaturated fats from plant-based sources include safflower, sunflower, corn, soybean, and cottonseed oils, and nuts.

A nut is actually a fruit composed of an inedible hard shell and a seed, which is generally edible. In common usage and in a culinary sense, a wide variety of dried seeds, like almonds and Brazil nuts, are commonly referred to as "nuts." In a botanical context, "nut" implies that the shell does not open to release the seed, like pecans and (some) pistachios.

Omega-3 fats are types of poly-unsaturated fats that have heart-protective benefits and are associated with lowering inflammation in the body. Types of Omega-3 fats include cold-water fish, such as salmon, tuna, herring, and anchovies. Plant-based sources of omega-3 fats include flaxseeds, chia seeds, and walnuts.

Saturated Fats Are Often Not So Good

Saturated fats are generally solid or waxy at room temperature, and with the exception of tropical oils (coconut oil, etc.), are derived mostly from animal products. Taking in too much saturated fat is linked with raising levels of "bad" LDL cholesterol, which can cause an increase in internal inflammation—never a good thing.

Healthy adults should limit their saturated fat intake to no more than 10 percent of total calories. For a person ingesting two thousand calories a day, this would be twenty-two grams of saturated fat or less per day. If you have elevated LDL cholesterol levels, it is recommended to reduce your saturated fat intake to no more than 7 percent of total calories. Foods high in saturated fat include…

- Beef, pork, lamb, veal, and skin from poultry
- Hot dogs, bologna, salami, and other cured and/or smoked meats
- High-fat dairy products such as cream, ice cream, whole milk, 2% milk, cheese, 4% cottage cheese
- Butter, lard, bacon fat
- Tropical oils, such as palm, palm kernel, and coconut oil
- Baked goods, such as cookies, cakes, pastries, and croissants

Trans Fats

Trans fatty acids are formed when a liquid fat is changed into a solid fat through a process called hydrogenation. Many manufacturers use hydrogenated oils as an ingredient because it can modify the consistency of foods and extend their shelf life. Trans fats will raise levels of "bad" LDL cholesterol and decrease levels of "good" HDL cholesterol (see more on cholesterol below).

There are no safe levels of trans fat to eat each day, so try to avoid these entirely.

Even if a food is advertised as "trans-fat-free," it can still contain small amounts of trans fat. Therefore, avoid foods that list partially hydrogenated oils as ingredients. Sources of trans fat include:

- Solid margarine
- Shortening
- Powdered coffee cream, liquid flavoured coffee cream
- Convenience foods, such as certain brands of pre-packaged baked goods and snacks

Cholesterol

According to the American Heart and Stroke Association, "Cholesterol is a waxy substance produced by your body to build cells and make vitamins and various hormones." While not inherently bad, too much cholesterol can pose a problem.

Cholesterol is derived from two sources. Your liver makes all the cholesterol your body requires to fulfill its everyday functions; the remainder comes from foods ingested that are made from animal sources. Meat, poultry, and dairy products all contain dietary cholesterol.

These same foods are also high in saturated and trans fats. These fats can cause your liver to manufacture more cholesterol than it otherwise would. For some people, this added production means their normal cholesterol level can rise to an unhealthy level.

Some tropical oils, such as palm, palm kernel, and coconut oil, contain saturated fats that can increase bad cholesterol. These oils are often found in commercially prepared baked goods.

Why Cholesterol Matters

Cholesterol circulates in the blood. As the amount of cholesterol in your blood increases, so does the risk to your health. High cholesterol contributes to a greater risk of cardiovascular diseases, such as heart disease and stroke. That's why it's important to have your cholesterol tested, so you can know and understand your levels.

The two types of cholesterol are LDL cholesterol, which is bad, and HDL, which is good. Too much of the bad kind or not enough of the good kind can increase the possibility that cholesterol will slowly build up in the inner walls of the arteries that feed the heart and brain.

More about LDL, HDL, and Triglycerides

Cholesterol can join with other substances to form a thick, hard deposit on the inside of the arteries. This can narrow the arteries and make them less flexible—a condition known as atherosclerosis. If a blood clot forms and blocks one of these narrowed arteries, a heart attack or stroke can result.

When it comes to cholesterol, remember to check, to change, and to control.

That is:

- **Check** your cholesterol levels. It's key to know your numbers and assess your risk.

- **Change** your diet and lifestyle to help improve your levels.

- **Control** your cholesterol, with help from your doctor if needed.

High cholesterol is one of the major controllable risk factors for coronary heart disease, heart attack and stroke. If you have other risk factors, such as smoking, high blood pressure, or Diabetes, your risk increases even more.

The more risk factors you have and the more severe they are, the higher your overall chance of having a bad episode or even a disease.

If your cholesterol levels are normal, limit your intake to no more than three hundred milligrams per day. If you have been diagnosed with high cholesterol, limit your intake to less than two hundred milligrams per day.

Limit These Nutrients

Total Fat 12g	18%
Saturated Fat 3g	15%
Trans Fat 3g	
Cholesterol 30mg	10%
Sodium 470mg	20%

Example: In a daily diet, the food in this example contributes 18 percent Daily Value (DV) of total fat, 15 percent DV of saturated fat, 10 percent DV of cholesterol, and 20 percent DV of sodium. In addition, it contains three grams of trans fat, for which a daily value percentage can't be calculated.

You don't need to memorize definitions for nutrient claims, such as "reduced fat," "light," "non-fat," and "low-fat." Just compare the daily value percentage for total fat to see which food product is lower or higher.

Most packaged foods now list their components. And, since cholesterol is found in animal-based foods, all you have to do is monitor the amount of "flesh" you eat (this includes dairy, which comes from animals).

Milk Alternatives

While we are accustomed to eating products made from soy, like tofu, which is essentially a cheese made from soy milk, a new industry based on manufacturing non-dairy milks and cheeses has appeared to address the needs of individuals attempting to avoid animal-based dairy products.

Over the past few years, a number of non-lactose, faux-dairy products have been developed. You can now go into most coffee shops and order one of these non-dairy alternatives in your latte. Plant-based milk alternatives can be made from legumes such as soy, or grains (oats, quinoa, rice, or teff), nuts (almond or coconut), or seeds (flax or hemp).

If you suffer from lactose intolerance, or if you just want to avoid animal products, plant-based milks provide an excellent alternative.

The base component of these alternative dairy sources will have some effect on the flavour of the milk. My personal preference is coconut milk because it offers sweetness without a heaviness or nuttiness factor. My friends swear by almond or cashew milk for a rich addition to coffee.

Besides non-dairy, milk-based cheesiness, nutritional yeast can create a creamy texture and a cheesy, nutty flavour in some foods. It can sub for cheese and add a bit of decadence or richness to a dish.

Nutritional yeast is made by pasteurizing and drying out *saccharomyces cerevisiae*, the yeast strain used to bake bread, *Bon Appetit* explains. The drying process deactivates the yeast (which means it won't be any use to you when baking), extracts the nutrients, and breaks down the yeast into flakes reminiscent of fish food. Livestrong indicates that this food is rich in B vitamins, supports a healthy immune system, is a good source of fibre, and can lower cholesterol levels.

It's Not Difficult - It Just Requires a Bit of Explanation!

One of the statements I hear most often with new clients is "I've always had problems with food." This is really vague and often leads (after a great deal of questioning!) to the statement "I guess I'm just lazy and we can't really do much about that." I convince them that it is only fear of the unknown. One of the hardest things to learn with food intake is not to starve yourself. In fact, with forethought and planning, we may actually find that you're not eating enough! Given proper food combinations, you can eat *more*! Doesn't that sound great?!

Macronutrients and Micronutrients

In a very simplified explanation, macronutrients are the major players of the body—carbs for energy production, protein for muscle building, and fats for hormonal balance.

Micronutrients are specialists working on smaller but very important tasks, protecting us from disease, keeping glandular production up, improving digestion. Some examples of micronutrients are zinc, manganese, iron, and copper.

Unless you're a trained naturopath or other type of doctor, chances are you won't be able to gauge if you're missing one or more specific micronutrients. Be that as it may, if you eat a variety of good food, fruits, vegetables, and nuts/seeds, and if you eat the right quantities of the macronutrient foods, you are likely to be getting sufficient micronutrients. Only through blood work or other testing methods, supervised by your doctor, will you be able to tell what might be missing.

If you prefer your mashed potatoes white, peel them, but know that the peel contains about 40 to 50 percent dietary fibre and has been considered as a new source of fibre and are a source of vitamins like riboflavin, ascorbic acid, folic acid, and vitamin B6. In addition to these, potato peels are a rich source of phenolics, which have been shown to bound carcinogens and are reported to have anti-carcinogenic properties.[4.]

But, let's face it, on fries or wedges or baked, the peel is delicious, and...

Bonus! Recipe:

Wash, dry, then peel your potato in a bowl, drizzle your peels with olive oil, sprinkle with the herb flavouring of choice (salt, garlic, rosemary, thyme, chili powder), then bake at 425 for 15-20 minutes. You'll not want to buy potato chips in a store ever again!

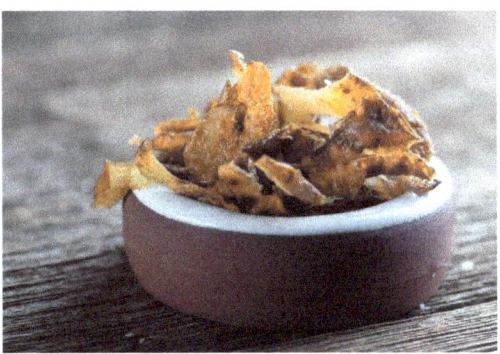

Blanching

Certain nutrients may also be lost during the blanching process. In fact, the greatest loss of nutrients can occur at this time.

Blanching takes place prior to freezing, and involves placing the produce in boiling water for a very brief time—usually a few minutes and sometimes only seconds, like green beans. This process kills any harmful bacteria and prevents the loss of flavour, colour, and texture. Yet it also results in a marginal loss of water-soluble nutrients, such as B-vitamins and vitamin C. This doesn't apply to frozen fruit, which doesn't often undergo blanching.

The extent of nutrient loss varies depending on the type of vegetable and length of blanching. Generally, losses range from 10 to 80 percent, with averages around 50 percent. This should not dissuade anyone from buying fresh, local, in-season vegetables and blanching them prior to consuming.

That being said, some research also suggests that frozen produce may retain its antioxidant activity despite the loss of water-soluble vitamins.

Nutrients in Both Fresh and Frozen Produce May Decline During Storage!

How Fresh Are Your Vegetables?

It is a given that fresh fruits and vegetables are full of vitamins, minerals, and antioxidants (micronutrients), all of which can improve our overall health. Eating more fruits and vegetables may even help protect against heart disease.

Given climate and seasonality, in many parts of the world, fresh produce isn't always available, and frozen varieties are a convenient and reasonable alternative, even though the nutritional values may vary. This latter point is predicated on harvesting, processing, and transportation methods.

Once they reach the supermarket, fruits and vegetables may spend an additional one to three days on display. They're then stored in people's homes for up to seven days before being eaten.

The vitamin C in fresh vegetables begins to decline immediately after harvesting and continues to do so during storage. However, although vitamin C can easily be lost during storage, antioxidants like carotenoids (which affect pigments in plants) and phenolics (critical in plant development) may actually increase. This is possibly due to continued ripening, and may be seen in some fruits.

Should you worry about this? Likely not. Eating fresh fruits and vegetables post-harvest is still far preferable to not eating them at all.

If you're not planning on eating fresh produce within a couple of days of bringing it home, you may wish to opt for either postponing the purchase or using frozen. Studies that demonstrate higher levels of certain nutrients in frozen are comparing the items to those that have been sitting on your counter or in the fridge for a number of days. For example, frozen peas or spinach may have more vitamin C than these same items purchased at the supermarket that have been stored at home for several days.

Frozen vs. Fresh

Concerned about the nutrition lost when using frozen versus fresh fruit or vegetables? In general, studies have shown that freezing can preserve nutrient value, and that the nutritional content of fresh and frozen produce is similar.

Fruits and vegetables that will be frozen are generally picked at peak ripeness, when they're the most nutritious. Once harvested, the vegetables are often washed, blanched, cut, frozen, and packaged within a few hours. Fruits can be treated with ascorbic acid (a form of vitamin C) or have some form of sugar added to prevent spoilage.

Usually, no chemicals are added to fresh produce before freezing. Generally speaking, freezing helps retain the nutrient content of fruits and vegetables. However, some nutrients begin to break down when frozen produce is stored for more than a year.

Levels of vitamin A, carotenoids, vitamin E, minerals, and fibre are similar in fresh and in frozen produce. And considering our discussion on blanching, that part of the process does not negatively affect the healthiness of your fruit or veggies.

Studies comparing supermarket produce with frozen varieties—such as peas, green beans, carrots, spinach and broccoli—found the antioxidant activity and nutrient contents to be similar.

Anecdotally, for some fruits, freeze-drying resulted in higher vitamin C content when compared to fresh varieties.

Treating Fresh Produce for Preservation

Most of the fruits and vegetables we buy are harvested by hand, with a smaller amount being harvested by machinery. And most fresh fruits and vegetables are picked before they are ripe. This allows them time to fully ripen during transportation, which is good for business! However, this method also gives fruits less time to develop a full range of vitamins, minerals, and natural antioxidants. This is not necessarily good for you!

There are many treatment methods used to preserve fruits and vegetables before they get to the grocery store. These methods keep the food fresh as it is packaged and transported.

Although many types of fresh produce travel across the world to get to your table, buying local and seasonal when possible is optimal for your health and safety. Having said that, who doesn't love strawberries and melons in February…?

In North America, fruits and vegetables may spend anywhere from three days to several weeks in transit before arriving at a distribution center. And the US Department of Agriculture (USDA) states that some produce, such as apples and pears, can be stored for up to twelve months under controlled conditions before being sold.

How Fresh Produce is Treated – The Good, the Bad

During transportation, fresh produce is generally stored in a chilled, controlled atmosphere and may be treated with chemicals to prevent spoilage. These types of treatments vary in efficacy and in safety but have been deemed safe by various US and Canadian government agencies. These treatments provide a broad range of preservation requirements like delays in ripening, preservation of colour and texture, inhibiting microbial growth and ethylene biosynthesis, reducing browning and the incidence of postharvest disease/decay, and potentially improving fruit colour and texture.

The Dirty Dozen and The Clean Fifteen

The Environmental Working Group (EWG) just released its 2022 "Dirty Dozen" list, which shows the fruits and veggies most contaminated with residues from pesticides according to research by the USDA. [5]

Here's the EWG's full list of the 2022 Dirty Dozen rankings:

1. Strawberries
2. Spinach
3. Kale, collard & mustard greens
4. Peaches
5. Pears
6. Nectarines
7. Apples
8. Grapes
9. Bell & Hot Peppers
10. Cherries
11. Blueberries
12. Green Beans

The results of years of ingesting these chemicals have not been studied enough to call it safe. Despite the fact that it is a pain, unless you've purchased your fresh produce directly from your organic farmer, really washing your fruits and veggies should be obligatory.

Here's the full list of 2022's Clean Fifteen; that is those fruits and vegetables that are mostly free from chemical and treatment residue:

1. Avocadoes
2. Sweet corn
3. Pineapple
4. Onions
5. Papaya
6. Sweet peas (frozen)
7. Asparagus
8. Honeydew melon
9. Kiwi
10. Cabbage
11. Mushrooms
12. Cantaloupe
13. Mangoes
14. Watermelon
15. Sweet Potatoes

If you notice, most of these require peeling or cooking of the skin/shell. In other words, wash your vegetables and fruit when you bring them home from the grocery store.

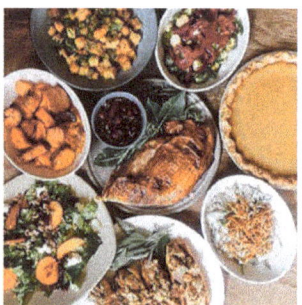

Shopping

Shopping for groceries can be done two ways: purchasing sufficient food to last a sustained period or buying daily for the next twenty-four hours. This latter is lovely, but neither exactly practical nor sustainable. Considering the pace and structure of my life, I prefer buying for a one- or two-week period, which allows for better efficiency.

If you buy at a larger grocery store, spend more time on the outer aisles—fresh produce, breads, meats, fish, and frozen vegetables are almost always on the perimeter. The inner aisles are reserved for more processed foods, canned goods, pastas, sugars, and fats (also known as "cookies").

Some foods, such as tuna, sardines, beans of various types, elements for soups and stews, are usually canned, and there is a regular need for these. But always examine the ingredients list of a tin and learn which have preservatives or chemicals. My general rule: if an ingredient has a number in it or if I can't pronounce it, I won't buy it!

If you can find a small and local grocer for emergency stops, a butcher for specialty meats, a fishmonger (often hard to find, but worth the effort), you will improve the quality of what you're eating and enjoy the experience even more!

Setting Yourself Up for a Good Week!
Meal Prep and Why I Love my Workplace Microwave!

Sundays when I'm at home are commitment afternoons for me. I prepare six daily meals and freeze them. It's become a science of chemistry, and a Zen experience (imagine eating this!) all at the same time.

Oven on, regular potatoes and sweet potatoes washed and ready, baking pans lined with parchment or foil; then carbs in the oven, rice cooker set and on; freezer containers set out in six rows. Then, a pan for chicken, one for ground turkey, and another for fish. When the carbs are ready, the protein goes into the oven and the ground turkey is sautéed with veggies and curry or smoked paprika or chipotle or cumin, or whatever flavour suits me. Once everything is cooked, the scale comes out, carbs are weighed and put into meal containers, followed by the same process with protein, selected veggies for each. Final step is various flavours—lemon pepper, mixed herb and spice blends, salsa of various types, pico de gallo. Each meal is seasoned and modified individually to provide variety and interest. Seal containers, label with contents, and arrange in the freezer.

Of late, in an attempt to cut down my meat consumption, I've been adding a lot of dried legumes to my diet. The only difference is a bit more prep, in that I have to start the soaking process the night before I plan to eat that meal.

We never really know what we're going to want to eat on a given day, so I don't preselect. Rather, I pick out what I want on the day I'm going to eat it.

Why only six containers? When I'm prepping the other days of the week, I'm also making myself something totally different to eat for Sunday night dinner, a bit of a treat. Or we might have takeout—a real treat!

Do you have to do this? No! This is an example only.

But it answers this question: I have a busy schedule! How am I supposed to organise?

Involve the Kids. Let's address the conundrum of how to feed your kids as well as yourself. Make them a part of the prep, let them chop and set up. Also, choose a couple of meals for them to enjoy and get them to prepare those. Choose a meal or two for nights when everyone is together at home enjoying a family meal. What a wonderful opportunity to teach them how to cook and eat properly! What a gift for them!

Now, I don't have any children, but I do have a husband who isn't as nutritionally driven as I am, and while he mostly deals with my lifestyle, working together and making something we can both enjoy has made for a healthier and happier mealtime experience.

Does this mean no social life? Let me tell you about my friends' wedding, when I was one week from a bodybuilding competition. It was a challenge, and despite the best efforts of the bride and groom to accommodate me, I broke the rules. Does this mean I should not have gone? Of course not! Our social life is an important part of our voyage. What I should have done was to have a small meal or even a snack before arriving, stayed away from the hors d'oeuvres and dessert table, and perhaps just had the main course. But, I danced the night away and had a wonderful time.

And that is also what keeps us youthful: enjoying the company of others, good food, good conversation. Simply plan ahead to be safe and help you stick to your plan.

Does this mean no alcohol? No, it does not.

I have chosen not to drink, but there is no reason for most of you to avoid the occasional cocktail. But if there is a weight loss period in your plans (and perhaps even longer term), let me pose this question: "Is the caloric, non-nutrient value worth the effect of the alcohol?" I have found that a well thought out mocktail adds pleasure to the event, and not to my waistline. Also, it's not just the calories contained in alcoholic drinks, it's the deleterious way that alcohol affects our body's ability to metabolize food. Here's how…

There are almost 155 calories in one twelve-ounce can of beer, and 125 calories in a five-ounce glass of red wine. A night out with several drinks can lead to consuming a few hundred extra calories. Drinks that have mixes, such as fruit juice or soda, contain even more calories. (By comparison, a recommended afternoon snack should have between 150 and 200 calories.)

When you drink, the first thing used as fuel for the body is the alcohol, meaning that the other nutrients you've consumed either *wait* or end up as *weight*, and are stored as adipose tissue, which is fat.

Again, the calories in alcohol are simple carbs, high in calories, and if you're not burning them, you're keeping them around. (It's not called a "beer gut" for nothing.) We can't choose where all that extra weight ends up, but the body tends to accumulate fat in the abdominal area.

Let's face it, after a few beverages, most of us put the other dietary restrictions away. It's really hard to say no to delicious treats when you're drinking. Studies suggest that alcohol can actually trigger hunger signals in the brain, leading to an increased urge to eat more food.

Finally, alcohol stresses the stomach and the intestines, which can lead to decreased digestive secretions and movement of food through the GI tract. Digestive secretions are an essential element of a healthy gut, as they break down food into the basic macro- and micro-nutrients that are absorbed and used by the body. Alcohol intake of any level can lead to impaired digestion and absorption of these nutrients.

For the Guys: It has long been acknowledged that alcohol intake can affect levels of hormones in the body—especially testosterone, which plays a role in many metabolic processes, including muscle formation and fat burning. Low testosterone levels may predict the prevalence of metabolic syndrome in men.

Metabolic syndrome is characterized by…

- high cholesterol
- high blood pressure
- high blood sugar levels
- high body mass index

Plus, lower testosterone levels may affect quality of sleep—especially in older men.

Back in the supermarket, I'd like to say this - with the exception of meat, the words "best before" do **not** indicate that at midnight on a certain date, the food will kill you. Global estimates indicate that one third of all food produced is wasted.

Very often, items are on sale as they get close to their expiry or sell-by date. In my opinion, these are still usable in soups, parts of a salad, or cooked immediately. This stops waste, feeds you well, and pads your wallet.

Chapter 6

Who is Your Guiding Star?

On any voyage, the navigator always has, at minimum, the North Star—or, in the Southern hemisphere, the Southern Cross to guide them.

What or who do you have?
What or who is it that leads us?

For those with a more spiritual or religious leaning (or training), this may be an easy question to answer. Your God or divine being, Ka, Chi, force, higher power, or creator may be the main guiding, driving, or comforting force. When looking for the answers to life's big questions, seeking solace when times get tough, searching for guidance when challenges are present—these are all occasions when we look to a greater power for help. We are reassured and supported in our hearts and in our souls by having a source of direction to guide us on our path.

Even those who are atheist or agnostic may still have a set of principles or philosophic/spiritual teachings to which they conform. Others may have a group of people, a crew, or individuals they trust implicitly, and who embody a set of behaviors with which they agree and to which they adhere. This might be a 12-Step group or even a Landmark Forum. Others might take exception to any group that conforms to what they perceive as a hive brain.

These behaviours or "credos" are the rules of conduct, proven to us over time, that can lead to a happier, more fulfilled life.

Perhaps it is not whom we ask, but that we ask. When difficulties or issues arise, making the time to step out of the problem, to examine it from all sides and come up with a plan of action, coolly—this is guiding yourself in the right direction.

As an example, the process of becoming sober, as I've said, and maintaining that sobriety, meant that I had to abandon certain relationships.

And conversely, there are those who have left us whose model lives on.

In the mid-seventies, I briefly had a good friend who I later ostracised through my own bad habits. I was a hairdresser—unisex, as was the trend in those days. This friend referred her father to me, because he was looking for a good "barber" (I did bristle slightly at that, but really, you're cutting hair, let's not get caught up in words). And on the first day, first appointment, in walks this suited business guy, and so began a decade-long relationship. Every four weeks, Henry sat in my chair and revealed more of his life to me. He enjoyed working out and had done so for years, even spearheading the building of a new YMCA in that city. He was retired and so was attending university, studying Latin, Greek, and the history of those two languages. In high school, I had studied six years of Latin, and loved the language. Henry rode his bike to and from school every day, often participating in longer charity rides. Although I also enjoyed working out, I hadn't yet discovered the joys of cycling. Henry was a man I admired, and I swore I would be like him someday. And here I am, approaching seventy, loving the gym and cycling, planning eventually to go back to school. Guess what I'll be studying?!? Henry is long gone, but he is still with me, daily, serving as a guiding star!

As I have tried to show throughout this book, life is a series of choices, and only we can make these decisions. First *if* and then *how* we choose to examine and face life's challenges are what is important, not the guiding force we employ to get us there.

While I personally have what I see as a strong relationship with my Creator, I still need to tackle a challenge with a piece of paper—a list of pros and cons, and perhaps the opinions of several trusted friends (my crew, as it were). It can often be too easy to get caught up in the emotional drama of an issue. Take the time to think it through and work out the benefits/detractions of various solutions before embarking on that particular change of direction.

Chapter 7

Mentorship and Support

Who will crew your ship?
Who teaches you? Do you need help?

Is our resistance to change an issue of ego? As I began my voyage, I thought I could manage most things on my own, only to discover that I could not! This was a **very** difficult lesson to learn.

It has been my experience that when I listen to trusted advisors, things go well, and when I storm ahead unheeding of guidance, the results are very unsatisfactory. People are put onto our paths in order to teach us, just as we are put onto the paths of others. Although we don't always understand or appreciate it (Heaven help those whose job has been to teach *me* patience and tolerance…), we are better off when we are open to accepting the lessons of our mentors.

As we move forward in our journey and acquire new habits, new joys, and new disciplines, we will have need of guidance. Like any new endeavour, there are those with experience and knowledge willing to take our hands and help us. These are the crew members for your craft called *life*.

While it is possible that most captains have learned every other job on the ship in their rise to leadership (any experienced manager should be able to do the job of the people they are leading), as a neophyte you would do well to select each member of your crew wisely and cautiously.

Who Is Your Crew?

Let's start with those who will be your right-hand people, the real life equivalent of the…

Mate (or First Mate, First Officer): Somehow, nerd that I am, I think of Spock in this role, and would give this position to one of two types of individuals. What's called for here is wisdom and the ability to look at an issue from all sides, then suggest the best plan of action. If you are part of a religious or spiritual fellowship, this may fall to your pastor/rabbi/imām/sponsor. Or this can also be the trusted best friend, the person who will look out for your best interests from all angles and at all times.

Now, let's say that you aren't a person with a religious background. There are still those people you know you can turn to in any situation. These may be family members, or someone who has always been around (whether you appreciated them or not!). I have to admit that I have a handful of people who have driven me crazy for years—they called when I didn't want them to, they showed up at events and talked to me when I wanted to float through the evening or just be left to my own devices. And to be honest, there were times when I was just too drunk to want to talk anyway. But now, years later, these pests, still in my life, still knowing me better than most, have proven to be the kind of honest, thoughtful, loyal, and yes, *pushy* people I appreciate—and I am grateful that they stuck around. Anybody have one or two of those?

In times of need or confusion, these are the people who will be there to help! Ask them aboard!

Second Mate (or Second Officer): I would suggest that this is the person most familiar with the methods you plan to employ to achieve your *physical* changes. This is your personal trainer, health or other type of coach, ballet or other dance master, yoga instructor, kinesiologist, etc. As with any new skill, search out the best teacher or guru that you can, then listen and learn. And don't stop at one! There can be several people in this role. Let me explain.

The overall scope of this book about the voyage, is to create a lot of change in a number of different facets of your life. Feel welcome to include any professional with a unique specialty that suits your needs. You'll then need a second, who knows about another area you've chosen to explore. You may need guidance for your overall physical fitness, a personal trainer of a sort, but if you then add running to your mix, you may need someone who is an experienced runner to help. Perhaps after running for a few months, the little voice in your head says, "Try a marathon." You might want to get a marathoner to support you with their experience in the field. (This may or may not be the person who is already your running mentor, depending on the level of expertise needed.)

As my own journey has unfolded, I hired a personal trainer (several over the years), then my needs evolved to include a trainer specifically for competitive bodybuilding. Recently, with the advent of COVID-19 and my discovery of the thrill of triathlon work, I have recognized the need for a running coach, a cycling coach, and a swimming coach. I now have to merge all these various types of training into a coach for triathlons. This individual will help me put the three together and teach me how to deal with the extra challenge of the transition between each skill, as well as completing the entire event.

Bosun (or Third Mate/Third Officer): Here I'm going to address something that most of us have not been trained to understand: money management. Many of us were never formally taught about money and, given our goal of achieving a longer, more active life, we need to use our funds as wisely as possible. So, I would suggest that if you do not already have a trusted financial person to set goals, examine where your money is going and how to optimize growth, you should seriously consider doing so. What I'm noticing, due largely to the pandemic, but also as a result of aging along with my peers, is that money is a huge issue for a great many of us.

Consider the fact that our lives may be lengthened by the new science of gerontology (by "new," I mean the proliferation of research into the causes and possible therapies for aging or anti-aging). Evidence is pointing to life expectancy increasing by a decade or more as we approach the middle of this century, 2050. And it's not so unthinkable that some of us will live long enough to reap the benefits of this work (*Ageless: The New Science of Getting Older Without Getting Old*, Andrew Steele). *Great news,* you say, *but how will I afford to live so long?*

Although it seems that there have already been significant changes in terms of career trajectories, with many of us having second and even third careers, we'll all have to focus on longer-term investments to support our longer lives (starting early, of course). Right now, many of us will need to take a cold, hard look at our relationship to money and start charting a course to improve our return on our investments so we can enjoy our lives during those additional years.

Chief Engineer (or "The Doctor Is In"): Since the job of the engineer is to know the workings of the ship, this role might be the best position for your family practitioner. As a generalist, your doctor is going to be your first advisor to address any ongoing physical issues. I believe that by embarking on this voyage, you will be making the most of your "healthspan," increasing your chances of a long and pleasurable life. However, there are still those issues (like the present onset of COVID-19 or any future occurrences of similar illnesses) that may need the advice of a doctor (not to mention the accidents, incidents, episodes, and even genetic issues which might pop up.)

As new therapies appear to help us improve on life quality, having a doctor with whom you can have real conversations will become more important (but still, please have your questions written down when you go for the visit. Nothing worse for me than leaving the appointment and thinking "damn, I forgot to ask about *xyz*"). Remember, your general practitioner is the gatekeeper to the specialists you may need.

Augment Your Crew

Who else do you want on board with you? Is there a family member, a friend, a co-worker? Start a list of your own—think of what roles they might play as you begin or continue your voyage.

A note about mutual responsibility: The fact that these people are giving you their time, energy, and help is a strong indicator that you may be asked to be a crew member on their ship, in addition to being captain of your own. Reciprocity is a beneficial, necessary, and critical facet of life. So, whenever you get help, even from a paid professional, think about how you can return the gift. The spirit of giving will bring more back to you, and consequently, to your journey.

Chapter 8

Smooth Sailing and the Danger of Complacency

Isn't it wonderful just letting the breeze push us along?

Smooth sailing just feels soooo good, right? When the wind is in our sails, not a cloud in the sky, gentle lapping waves, and we're relaxing and headed in the right direction, it seems like the best of all possible worlds. Why bother toiling when destiny seems to be doing all the work for us? As a life, a business, or a relationship begins to build, the natural urge is to put the requisite effort into the growth process. So it is with the changing of habits. Once the initial momentum has been achieved, coasting can feel appropriate, even freeing. And then? Attention to detail falls off, motivation flags, energy is re-directed, and so on.

But it bears remembering that the work necessary for accomplishment is what can make the result that much sweeter for us.

Let's examine this.

If we look at travel quest books, such as Homer's *Odyssey* or Voltaire's *Candide* or *All for the Best* (1759), we find that our travellers have many more difficulties dealing with laziness and taking the easy way than they have when dealing with adversity. Odysseus and his men encountered the Land of the Lotus Eaters, whose inhabitants were enchanted by the power of the Lotus, then chose to remain there, abandoning their quest to go home. Why? Because it was easier than the struggle involved in the return to the lives they'd left behind.

Candide, after all his adventures had hardened him to the world, saw perfection in a small plot of ground and the corresponding opportunity to make his garden grow. He understood fully that labour can bring about a tranquility far more significant than the ease offered by great wealth. After travelling the world to find his happiness, he has found it within. This was also true for two little girls we all know: Alice and Dorothy.

Shakespeare and others spoke of life *not* being a state of ease, comfort or pleasure—not, in fact, a "bed of roses."

So, what does this all mean for us? If life is too easy, or if the desire to continue our future quests becomes less important than our present, we can often abandon our goals.

For example, having visited the doctor and being told I was looking at incipient Type 2 Diabetes *and* high blood pressure, I decided I needed to change my physical state. I acquired some diet books, shopped for a much healthier pantry, started walking and exercising. My goal was to lose twenty pounds and hopefully halt the onset of the two impending, life-altering diseases.

A month went by and—*hooray*—I lost ten pounds. So now, I guess, it's OK to eat something not allowed in my diet. And then, the next morning when I woke up it was pouring rain, so I pulled the covers over my head and didn't exercise. And then, the next day, I was busy, and so too the next, and gradually I saw that the scale had started to reverse. (This is actually what I did! Sound familiar?)

When this happened, I was left with the choice to get back on my boat or stay where I was. As it turned out, I did not get on my boat, and I put the ten pounds back on. And then I added another fifteen.

Another scenario: I started this diet three weeks ago, I've lost twelve pounds, and so far, I'm very happy with it. Since I'm going out with friends tonight and I haven't seen them for three weeks, I might have a little treat. Right? Seems innocent enough…

Then, next weekend, I'm seeing a different group of friends, so another treat might be OK. Soon, every weekend is a reason to have a treat. Shockingly, the results seem to have slowed down—or worse, I've gained weight.

In high school, fifty years or so ago, I was a straight-A student. But toward the end of Grade 10, I figured out that I was pretty hot stuff academically. So, while I farmed myself out to ghostwrite other students' papers, I also felt it was OK to party with friends or relax into dreams of what was going to happen as I got older. What I didn't do was pay attention to my own schoolwork—and, no surprise, my grades started to slip.

This has, at times, been a habitual pattern for me. When my hair salon became busy and popular, I stopped worrying about some of the details that had contributed to its growth. Each client was still cared for as well as I possibly could, but the management of the salon suffered (admittedly, my drinking and drug use also escalated during this period). I could not maintain stability in my business because I had other interests on my mind.

How many of us fall prey to the dreaded New Year's resolutions, which invariably are maintained for a few weeks—and by February, no resolution.

I think that complacency is the human trait that allows habits such as procrastination and sloth to get stronger. When I think that all is well and it's safe to rest on my laurels, my drive to push ahead is diminished.

I believe that languishing prevents future growth—the sense that I will just continue as I am, without worrying about the incremental changes that I need to continue the process of my life.

This stasis can affect us in so many ways.

Businesses lose their focus and fail. Relationships and partners can become so used to each other, it's easy to be distracted by irrelevant issues. When this happens, we can grow apart. When the extra effort to cherish each other disappears, then so can the relationship. Friendships that are based on "I'll call next week," but neither of you ever do, can put years between any future communication.

Can you name the one person you consider a good friend, but can't remember the last time you spoke? (And let's not try to fit social media in here. I'm talking face to face, even if it's Zoom.)

Taking a break, relaxing, putting your feet up is such a great feeling, isn't it? But the extra couple of minutes to reach out, to enrich your life, your relationships, opens doors otherwise unseen.

For many of us, the COVID-19 pandemic experience has been an eye-opener. From the outset, I made sure that I had what I needed to continue my own fitness journey. My basement was set up with rudimentary weights, resistance bands, and everything I now use to work with my clients who, due to lockdowns, have no access to the gym. Normally, when I am working and seeing clients at the gym, I set aside a specific time for my own workouts. But during the stay-at-home and lockdown situations, I've been working from my home office and sending video workouts to my clients. Departing from my regular, regimented gym timeframes—pre-work, lunch hours, post-work, peak periods—and scheduling and conducting Zoom workouts from home means distraction and disengagement. It is precisely this structural change that meant I could miss the odd workout, get busy with household chores, etc., in essence, falling prey to the very things I am paid to help my clients avoid.

I often listen to the great Les Brown, one of the world's most renowned motivational speakers. He speaks about being on one's deathbed surrounded by the hopes, dreams, and ideas offered during our lifetime. Why were some passed over or ignored? Will it be because of the external justifications we believed and the false stories we told ourselves? How will you feel?

When I consider all of the dreams of my childhood, youth, and adulthood, how many have remained in my heart and been brought to fruition?

This is not to suggest that we should constantly run toward whatever dream strikes us in the moment. But when our heart has told us that something is its desire, we should give it due consideration and, decision made, stick to the plan.

Ultimately, I think that complacency amounts to allowing habits such as procrastination and laziness to gather momentum. When I think that all is well, and it's safe to rest on my laurels, my drive to push ahead is diminished. It's just like the accumulation of dust bunnies; you must be on top of things all the time—or magically, they are floating across the floor.

So then, how to deal with this seemingly endless, self-defeating pattern?

I'm going to invite you to put aside a small piece of your time today to specifically conjure up some of your old dreams. Try to remember when you wanted to paint, take up karate, dance, sing, study—do some of these fit the voyage you're on right now? My fitness journey has led me to explore many facets of the fitness canon—ballet, swimming, body building, zip-lining. Not all of them grabbed me the way others did, but my entire existence is so much richer for having tried.

Chapter 9

Storms! Understanding Growth Through Adversity

Stormy weather is not *just* a great Lena Horne song—it's something we all have to face with regularity. Sometimes this inclement weather can be interpreted literally, and increasingly like the issues associated with climate change, which can destroy homes and cost lives. Storms can also take the form of emotional upheaval, the drama and pain that we can create so often in our own lives. And despite how hard these are to weather; they are very often that which makes us stronger.

Let me tell you about the greatest storm I've faced so far. I started drinking in my mid-teens—the usual house party stuff, if we don't mention the cocktails in my grandparents' basement when the only person at the party was me. By my mid-twenties, I was drinking steadily and heavily, and mixing a toxic blend of other substances.

I was a hard worker, dedicated to my hairdressing business, which I truly saw as and still believe to be an art form. I had reached the point where old friends, growing out of their party phase, were disappearing, and new friends with habits similar to mine were on the scene. I would regularly quit drinking to keep my business in place, get fit (working out obsessively as I drank), and getting out of whatever financial difficulties in which I found myself. Typically, a month or two would go by, and I would reward my good behaviour with a drink—"Sorry, my mistake"—drunk! And then, around October of 1989, I attended a party where I ran into someone I'd known since she was thirteen (she was now twenty). I cannot describe the look on her face, but her shock at seeing me so wasted rendered me speechless. So, did I decide to quit! *Hell no*!

It wasn't till the twenty-eighth of June 1990 that, having left an AA meeting and walking directly into a bar the night before, I was sufficiently defeated to call for help. Within two days, I was in another country, in a rehab facility, facing the storm and changing every aspect of my life.

So what do you think? Do our storms, when confronted, teach us more about our lives, about ourselves, and help us move further into a better version of ourselves?

The best swords are forged and re-forged, heated to white hot and beaten, cooled, and the process begun again. We are the same!

We face two choices when the bad thing occurs in our lives—we can either bemoan our fate, or we can learn the lessons. Yes, I believe that these lessons do come to us for a reason.

Do not think that I am lessening the effects of losing a loved one to a pandemic, a war, an act of nature! But when these things happen, we are called upon to find new strengths, to help others also dealing with these issues, to move forward.

I am thinking now of Lily Ebert, ninety-eight-year-old Holocaust survivor, who has recently been using TikTok to discuss her experiences to teach the story and the need for hope. As horrific as her story is, she has positivity to pass on.

Chapter 10

Which Fork in the Road? Determining If This Is What You Want

When I was in theatre school, studying in New York, I was given a copy of "The Road Not Taken," or as it is better known "The Road Less Travelled," by the great poet Robert Frost. I was forty at the time, choosing a second career that pulled at me so strongly that no one could convince me not to follow my dream. But, like many entering a new profession in mid-life, or at any age, fear of failure is never far, gnawing away at one's confidence. The chorus is familiar to all of us—that siren song about safety, security, paying the bills, and even encroaching age. A familiar companion, now known as impostor syndrome.

My experience, however, did teach me that the road had many twists and turns—dark areas and bright sunlight—and by taking this path, my path, the rewards would be countless.

> Robert Frost (1874–1963)
> Mountain Interval 1920 [6]
>
> **The Road Not Taken**
>
> *Two roads diverged in a yellow wood,*
> *And sorry I could not travel both*
> *And be one traveller, long I stood*
> *And looked down one as far as I could*
> *To where it bent in the undergrowth;*

Then took the other, as just as fair,
And having perhaps the better claim,
Because it was grassy and wanted wear;
Though as for that the passing there
Had worn them really about the same,

And both that morning equally lay
In leaves no step had trodden black.
Oh, I kept the first for another day!
Yet knowing how way leads on to way,
I doubted if I should ever come back.

I shall be telling this with a sigh
Somewhere ages and ages hence:
Two roads diverged in a wood, and I—
I took the one less travelled by,
And that has made all the difference.

Let's spend some time thinking about the roads you've chosen in your own life. Think about a few examples to show where or how you have made significant choices in the past. It would really help at this point if you wrote down your answers.

In school, did you choose the subjects about which you were truly passionate? Or did you choose those that would lead you to the "best career" or one that had the most "security"?

Did you or do you read what is suggested by teachers or friends, or do you wander the bookstore until a title grabs your attention (for pleasure or for a specific purpose)?

Do you prefer to order the same thing at your favourite restaurant, or do you go into new places and ask the server what they would suggest?

Do you follow others' advice, even if your gut suggests that you don't agree?

Do you listen to the same playlists because you know the words, and the emotions which might be evoked, or do you change the channel until you hear something new?

I don't wish to insinuate that you must always be changing, or that you should never listen to advice. I'm merely suggesting that changes might be in order at certain points in your journey.

Here's a story about my mother. Every change of season, there would be an intense week of housecleaning in preparation for the change in the weather. While this meant that there was a lot of cleaning and dusting, she also changed the appearance of the bedrooms and living areas, arranging the furniture differently, transforming the colour scheme of each room as the bed linens and/or curtains were all replaced. This was a way of welcoming the coming season, much the way that we would change the contents of our closets from summer clothes to winter attire and back again.

So, would you be comfortable with having the decor of your home completely changed on a regular basis, or would that actually make you uncomfortable?

It's not my place to dictate which of these choices is better. I have learned over the years, however, that adaptability to change is a very important trait. I do not mean to imply that chasing after every shining thing which appears in your path is right or even advisable. But I do feel that seeing change as a constant in our lives and being able to "go with the flow" serves us much better. This attribute will save us from the debilitating fear of the storm, and keep us from missing some of the incredible beauty ahead.

If I've learned anything during the COVID-19 pandemic, it is that nothing is actually under our control. And although this isn't always evident, sometimes, it becomes much more obvious. Circumstances help push us toward greater growth and change, or fear pushes us further back. We can make the choice.

On the other hand…

Chapter 11

Embracing and Accepting Your True Self

Looking at your life right now, what is it that makes you happy? What could a friend look at and say, yes, that defines you. Now let's look at what traits function in the same way. Do you consider yourself to be accepting of others? Do you have hope, some measure of faith (not necessarily in a higher power, but a belief in others, or in the world in general)? Would you say that you have courage in the face of adversity? How about honesty, patience, humility, willingness to grow, to learn, to go with the flow? Do you care about your fellow humans? Are you into charitable work (donations or time spent)? Do you live with integrity? Do people trust you? Are you self-disciplined and do you work to help others?

Who is the *true* you? You are an entire human being, the sum of the life experiences, events, decisions, procrastinations, influences, and all the other foundations that have created the person you are today. How you feel, your thought processes, your basic human self, is who we're talking about. The you that only *you* know.

Do you understand how we, paradoxes that we are, can pull ourselves in opposite directions and, in the process, make ourselves miserable? Self-reflection, finding out what our primary beliefs are, checking all of these against what we already know and then, working to alter that negativity, are essential tasks as we push toward our fountain.

There are many practices, including just running a business, which require taking an inventory. What inventory items do you personally have on the shelf? What are their past due dates? Are they in good working order?

Do you take the time to have a look and remove the bad stuff? Or are you a hoarder? What do you see as a heavy weight?

Think about and examine what you are observing. Look, inspect, analyse and really think about what you see. Certainly, as you've prepped for and begun this voyage, chosen how you would steer your vessel, you've encountered many inventory items of absolute personal value, and some that might be left behind.

The process of discovering which qualities most embody who we are allows us to see if they truly define us and determine whether they help or hinder us in our life plans. Consider: you want a flourishing career and the wealth that might bring, but you've been taught that money is the root of all evil. In this case, you may not allow yourself to acquire something which you desire and deserve because you remain conflicted about its value.

How about this: you can't trust anyone, but you want a relationship based on trust.

I don't know about you, but when I get into a tight spot, when things are particularly difficult, it is not always my noble, true self that I bring to meet these challenges. Rather, this is the very time that old habits, negativity, anger, fear—actually, this is the true culprit—show up to take control, often leaving me afterward with the "why didn't I react differently" question ringing in my mind.

Yes, I am the old guy on the bike explaining, often vehemently, why the bike lane is not for parking, even if it is to "just pick up your food order." I'm not proud of this behaviour, and I'm working on it. I should not be this guy, so what happens?

Growth is a long process—change of any kind is. And when we're troubled, the new training has a hard time keeping up. It is always best at times like this to take a moment and give yourself a few minutes, hours, days, or even weeks to reassess the situation. Remember who you are—your *true* self.

Easy? *No*! But like everything else in life, worth the effort.

Eventually, the new habits are strengthened, allowing the person you really are to truly flourish.

Embracing the Child Within

However you view this search for your inner being, the most fundamental and vulnerable part of yourself is critical to your next steps. Why is this important?

One of my core beliefs is this: as we've moved through our lives, we've been confronted with some form of trauma, usually inflicted by those who purport to or genuinely care about us. Tragically, the individuals who provoke this trauma are dealing with their own deficiencies and pain, and in their plan to protect us, they inadvertently teach us to fear. It's important to remember that the expectations of parents and family members are based on the paths they have taken and the perceived mistakes they've made. In order to protect us from stumbling in the same way, they endeavour to plan our lives, our expectations, even our futures. Most of us have been given some very intense "coding" that affects our social interactions, our worldview, and how we regard our own capabilities.

The issue here is to understand the lessons we've been taught that were imparted to protect us. Examine them closely and observe how you've internalized these lessons and how that perception has affected your view of yourself and subsequent actions.

By now, we've been on this journey for a while. We've had a chance to get more active, improve our nutrition and our sleep. We've looked at our sense of self, our relationships with the outside world. Doing an inventory of this type is essential as part of our lives. Carrying a lot of baggage as we get older is not an absolute necessity.

Importance of Core Values – Your Guiding Principles

Here's how my core values led me to my own voyage:

I have a firm conviction that we all, at certain points in our lives, face difficult trials. Resolving these, figuring out how to manage our way through these challenges, will serve to really help us understand who we are and what we believe in.

As someone who's evolved over the past few decades into a proponent of the kind of life we're discussing, I've had to make some difficult life choices. As an example, the process of becoming sober, as I've said, and maintaining that sobriety, meant that I had to abandon certain relationships. This action was taken not because I felt superior to these individuals—nor did I view them as "triggering" my addiction. But I did see them as being incompatible with the direction I knew my life had to take. What I believe is that if I want and need to be open and available to the change I am inviting into my being, then I need to clear space. I need to declutter if the *new* is going to flow in and replace the *old*, even though I have to know that it means taking some fairly uncomfortable steps.

Examine your core values and ensure that there's a match with the relationships you have that might be preventing you from achieving your goals or supporting your voyage.

However you view this search for your inner being, the most fundamental and vulnerable part of yourself is critical to your next steps. Why is this important?

Remembering Who You Are When Times Get Tough

I'd had what everyone (including me) agreed, was a brilliant career, culminating in a national role that was high-profile, well-paid and significant in the industry. As part of a cost-cutting measure, my division was closed and I was laid off. After five years in this position, to say I was devastated would be an understatement.

At the time, I believed I had no resources to deal with this trauma. I knew that I would have to figure out what was next for me, but for a long time, I was so deeply hurt, confused and shocked that I was unable to imagine moving on.

This wasn't the death of a loved one. No one I cared deeply about was sick and dying. I had my friends and family, and they were universally supportive. What was my distress? I was firmly caught up in the belief that "I am what I do," when the truth clearly was, and is "I am who I am, not what I do."

I'll admit that it took many months for me to recover and get down to finding other work and moving on from the loss of my former employment. I'd toyed with running away to another city or changing industries. I'd even pondered starting my own business.

But it wasn't until one of my dearest friends said to me, "Don't forget who you are," that I was able to see the way forward. I had forgotten who I was—a smart, capable, hardworking person who had only just turned forty and had much more life to experience.

Ultimately, I found work, kickstarted another phase of my career, and found new and different kinds of successes. And I did end up starting my own business, over twenty years later. I've often wondered what would have happened if I'd remembered who I was at that long-ago time in my life and had the confidence to trust myself and go out on my own. I'll never know the answer to that mystery, but I do know who I am. [7]

A Note on Social Media
or
Living in the Insta-World

It bears repeating that real life is not on Instagram, Facebook, TikTok, Pinterest or any other social media platform. While we don't actually believe these represent real life, we are definitely living in the age of FOMO (Fear Of Missing Out) and instant gratification. If we're on those platforms, it's extremely difficult not to expect immediate gratification from our everyday IRL (In Real Life) efforts.

We will not find our future in an instant. We have embarked on a journey that will take us our entire lifetime to complete. How exciting! Our only way is slow and steady, working hard to achieve our goals and thereby, our gratification. It's our life.

A Note on Joy with Marie Kondo

The popularity of Marie Kondo, who tells us to ask if an object sparks joy, can be equally useful in our lives. Do current relationships, your job, your Netflix queue serve you as you should be served? The trend toward the tiny house, even the subject of van life in the film (melancholic as it was) *Nomadland* points to the beauty of divesting ourselves of the material.

Marie Kondo

Late Life Changes

Sometimes, beginning anew is not our choice. What happens when we're in mid-life and we lose our job? What happens when we lose our spouse of many decades, who's always taken care of various things around the house that we haven't ever had to think about? We need to be able to figure out how we're going to manage, how to re-invent ourself, how we're going to succeed as a late-starter.

The changes these situations precipitate may seem insurmountable to us, as they can often be associated with emotional upheaval—even trauma. The lesson is to recover at your own pace, then tackle the issues that require learning new things.

Don't be afraid! Try to embrace the fear, and you may find it freeing to learn something new.

This question of figuring things out at any time in our lives is really one of identity. This is especially true as we age. We are certainly capable of learning how to do new things as we get older. We just need to remind ourselves of who we are.

Chapter 12

Last Thoughts

So finally, after all this time, the sight of land! What does this mean now? How do you feel? Ready to see the Grail for which you have worked all this time? The vessel has dropped anchor, and you board a small craft to take you closer to land. It's crowded, and the waves seem choppier than on the bigger boat, and when you get close enough to shore, you just have to jump, fully clothed, into the water. Your wet clothes make it harder to walk, not easier, and the sand is getting into your clothes and your boots, so that you almost have to crawl up the beach until enough of the water has drained out.

This is almost the end of the journey. There is a feeling of exhaustion and exhilaration all at once. You're almost there, almost there, keep going. Reach the end of the beach and then head into the bush, looking to the fountain.

Remember that there is a goal, a vision that you set months ago, a goal to find and be something. You have asked for help and gotten it. You have listened to advice and followed some of it. You have removed some old habits and gained some new ones. What does your life look like now? Take a moment to make a few notes about where you are in your life:

_____

_____

_____

_____

Now is the time for assessment. It's not enough to make the changes. You must consider whether, having achieved change, it actually pleases you. With the fountain just over the next ridge, sit down for some quiet contemplation. Look at yourself and think back on the you who began the journey. What qualities have you gained along the way? Are you more confident? Are you smiling more than previously? How are your relationships? Are there changes there? Some people may be gone from your life, if you were either not served by the other person, or if they felt you no longer suited them (It's a two-way street—we come into others' lives for a reason and we leave for a reason, without judgment). Jot down some answers to these questions:

_____

_____

_____

_____

_____

_____

_____

_____

_____

Many things have certainly changed for the better! You should be at a better weight and level of fitness than before. You have developed stronger relationships and have learned how to lead and how to support others. I would like to think that you are more clear-eyed, clear-headed, and have a greater sense of joy. Bravo! Brava! Brave one!

But…

Take the time again to look at any negatives which may have entered your life.

Many of us, in the drive to become fit, let this focus become the greatest driving force in our lives. Have you become overly regimented in your eating habits and the need to work out? Does a day of actual relaxation make you a bit crazy? Do you turn away from social engagements, either because of the food component or because your schedule is too strict to allow for it? Don't remove all the fun in your life in support of rigid self-discipline!

I have faced this myself! Many times, in my life, I have confused my priorities, and what seems to be the most important thing is truly not.

Does this happen in your life? At the beginning of my hairdressing career, I worked whatever hours needed to gain a clientele and build my business. Consequently, my relationship and my fitness both suffered.

Did relationships falter during your work-obsessed times? How many of us have let responsibilities in our jobs slide as we move through the joys of finding a new love, or while lovingly participating in the first year after the birth of a child? These are natural effects and countereffects. When we enter a new chapter of our development, it can take pride of place. The task here, then, is to remain mindful of this fact, and try to maintain balance.

Have you been too hard on yourself?

_____
_____
_____
_____
_____
_____
_____
_____
_____

Have you found that after trusting your crew and spending so much time with them that some family members, distant friends, even spouses, who were not part of the journey, have felt left out, and are even bewildered by who the new you is? Give them time, be kind but firm in the changes you have committed to; they will either return to the fold or they will leave your sphere. This is not a judgement of who you now are. We are not all meant to travel the same road permanently.

Here's another opportunity to review where you are in your life:

_____

_____

_____

_____

_____

_____

_____

_____

_____

A case in point: I had a boyfriend when I first got sober. He had actually been one of the catalysts of some of the changes in my life. I had hurt him with my drinking behaviour, and he gave me an ultimatum: "Get sober or I'm gone!" Our story progressed until eventually I did go to rehab and I was beginning the process of evolving. To my boyfriend, I was "changing." However, within two weeks, I heard "I want the old Walter back", because my behaviour was no longer predictable. Our relationship ended, as it needed to. We are still friends (of a social media type), but I will forever be grateful for that ultimatum, as it was the one more brick in the wall that forced sobriety, forced change into my life.

Chapter 13

Land Ho! The Fountain Is a Mirror

So here it is and here you are! The elusive Fountain of Life, your mirror. Gaze into it and see that there is no need to drink or bathe in the waters. What you see is a healthier, more youthful you. The worry lines on your face have smoothed out. They are not gone, but the easy smile, the look of calm resolution, have lessened them. Now that you're happier with yourself, the lines you see become a badge of honour, well-earned and a source of pride.

Your new, healthier body moves with more ease, more confidence. You have become one of the active, more athletic ones. You are not twenty, nor would you care to be, but movement is something to relish, no longer a source of fear of injury, or even embarrassment.

You are surrounded by those who think like you. This is not to say that you found a soulmate, but that loneliness is not crushing, and you are part of a community of your own making, the family you choose, not the one you are given.

Chapter 14

Epilogue

With all my heart, I hope that this has helped some of you make the changes you desire in your lives easier that it has nudged you to broaden your horizons and think, what else needs to happen?

I hope you find those activities that keep you smiling and progressing! Exercise is a wonderful thing. When you find the type that lights the fire, do what you can to keep the fire burning!

I hope you now view food as a wonderful gift to enjoy rather than a burden to deal with. Use it to enhance your life and your health, not as an emotional crutch or a wall to keep the world at bay.

Surround yourself with those people who will bolster you and celebrate you. Understand your responsibility to do the same for them. Joy and love will grow! Finally, please share your growth with me and your future friends. This link will hook you into a Facebook page for you:

Bon Voyage!

Wait, one more thing!
See the mountain just on the other side of the fountain?
What do you think is there, or just past it?
Let's find out!

Some extras

The "Mighty Mo" begins her second century as a swimming champion—*Los Angeles Times*.

From the Concept 2 Facebook page - Ninety-Year-Old Dean Smith Rows a World Record in 9:55.8.

10 Insightful Tips from People Who Prove It's Never Too Late

Addendum

Links to Complementary Articles

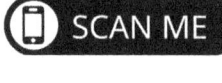

From the *Globe and Mail*: "Amplify: Forget Best-Before Dates—You're Never Too Old to Hit Your Stride," by Elizabeth Renzetti

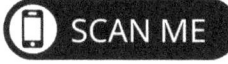

"Here's How I Finally Got Myself to Start Exercising," by Christine Carter, PhD

ideas.ted.com/heres-how-i-finally-got-myself-to-start-exercising

From the *Globe and Mail*: "How the Human Brain Can Turn Suffering into a Sense of Fulfilment," by Bruce Grierson

Acknowledgements

When I talk about the importance of the crew in this book, I really mean it.

My crew in getting this vessel out of port has been incredibly important to me and I could not have done this without their help. From the first thought forward, so many have pushed me along.

Maire Kushner, who has had my back throughout, offering advice or homemade biscotti. More than an editor, she has been a sounding board, a motivator, a good friend.

Matt Smith, business partner and the best workout partner!

Simon Tanenbaum, who helped me solidify the imagery for the book, and made me think about it from the other perspective—that of you, the reader.

Those mentioned in the book, Miss B, Mr. Davis, all the givers of nuggets of gold over the years, examples of drive, of the joy of living.

My family, the first teachers.

My clients over the years, who have trusted me when I wasn't sure I trusted myself.

To all of you sitting in basements all over the world, working on getting better, together.

Finally, to my husband, Martin, who has been there throughout, thick, and thin, sickness and health.

To the Creative Spirit in all of us, thank you!

Bibliography and Citations

1. S;, Volpi, E;Nazemi, R;Fujita. "Muscle Tissue Changes with Aging." Current opinion in clinical nutrition and metabolic care. U.S. National Library of Medicine, https://pubmed.ncbi.nlm.nih.gov/15192443/
2. "Body Mass Index (BMI) Calculator." Diabetes Canada Website. (Page 16) https://diabetes.ca/managing-my-diabetes/tools---resources/body-mass-index-(bmi)-calculator
3. "Protein for Fitness: Age Demands Greater Protein Needs" (Page 31)
   By Denise Webb, PhD, RD
   Today's Dietitian
   Vol. 17, No. 4, p. 16
4. Farvin, Sabeena, Alagarsamy, Surendraraj, Jacobsen, Charlotte
   Composition and health benefits of potato peel
   Potatoes: Production, Consumption, and Health Benefits (Page 43)
   2012/01/01
   196–227
5. "EWG's 2022 Shopper's Guide to Pesticides in Produce" (Page 49) https://static.ewg.org/upload/pdf/EWG_SG-2022_Guide.pdf
6. The Road Not Taken. Frost, Robert. 1920. Mountain Interval (Page 73) https://www.bartleby.com/119/1.html
7. Maire Kushner (Page 82)

About the Author

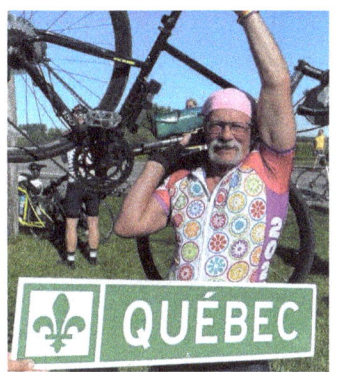

Walter Young is a professional trainer, avid athlete, and first-time author. Moved by experiences dealing with the drug and alcohol dependence of his youth, and building a career as a personal trainer in his mid-fifties, he aims to inspire others to invest in their physical well-being, regardless of age or skill.

At sixty-five, Walter continues to compete as a bodybuilder and to swim, run or bike four times a week. He has studied physical training, is certified in nutrition habit management and also enjoys weight training, running and athletic competitions. Walter lives in Toronto, with his husband, Martin and works as a Longevity Coach. You can reach Walter at @Coachwalterrenofit on Instagram, @Oldfitdude on TikTok, or on Facebook at facebook.com/walteryoung

About the Editor

Maire Kushner, a 35-year multi-disciplined veteran of the technology industry, held executive leadership positions in companies from start-ups to the Fortune500.

A writer by avocation, this first collaboration with Walter Young has enabled Maire to combine her passions for the culinary arts and physical fitness with her love of creative writing.

Maire is also a COVID-19 pandemic era cancer survivor and believes that her attention to good nutrition and physical activity are keys to her anticipated long and healthy future. She lives happily in Toronto with her partner, Marcus.

Reach out at: mairek@creativemarketinginsights.com

www.ingramcontent.com/pod-product-compliance
Lightning Source LLC
Jackson TN
JSHW070828261025
93175JS00002B/6